W9-CSR-149

A Dietitian's Journey to
Diabetes Prevention and Treatment

101 Ways to Control
Your Diabetes
By the Doctor's Dietitian

Susan B. Dopart, MS, RD, CDE

Photography Jeffrey M. Batchelor
Visual Design Ciara Christine

To all those who have the daily challenge
of blood glucose control and are committed
to better health and well-being

101 WAYS TO CONTROL YOUR DIABETES

Edition 1.1, First Printing: March 2017

SGJ Publishing
Santa Monica, California

Publisher's Cataloging-In-Publication Data
(Prepared by The Donohue Group, Inc.)

Names: Dopart, Susan B. | Batchelor, Jeffrey M., photographer. | Christine, Ciara, designer.
Title: 101 ways to control your diabetes by the doctor's dietitian : a dietitian's journey to diabetes prevention and treatment / by Susan B. Dopart, MS, RD, CDE ; photography, Jeffrey M. Batchelor ; visual design, Ciara Christine.
Other Titles: One hundred one ways to control your diabetes by the doctor's dietitian
Description: Edition 1.1. | Santa Monica, California : SGJ Publishing, [2017] | Includes bibliographical references.
Identifiers: ISBN 978-0-9860236-5-1 | ISBN 978-0-9860236-6-8 (ebook)
Subjects: LCSH: Diabetes--Diet therapy. | Diabetes--Prevention. | Diabetes--Treatment.
Classification: LCC RC662 .D66 2017 (print) | LCC RC662 (ebook) | DDC 616.4/620654--dc23

Table of Contents

ACKNOWLEDGEMENTS

I am grateful for all those who help make our books possible.

To my clients who are continually curious, want the most up-to-date information, and struggle with the daily task of managing diabetes. I am thankful for the trust they place in me to help them along their journeys.

I want to thank all who provided edits and guidance on the flow and readability of the book, including Barbara Olivo, Joseph Dopart, Suzanne Hollander, MS, RD, CSP, and Pamela Lee, MPH, RD, CDE.

I am thankful for Debra Lesin Elliott, FNP, CDE, BC-ADM, who tirelessly provided help and edits for accuracy and clarity of the book and the medication chapter. Her support of my books and projects goes beyond what a person could hope for in a colleague and friend.

Many thanks to Omar Aziz and Ciara Christine for their countless hours in design, and their vision for the look and concepts provided in this book. Their dedication to our projects is much appreciated.

Special thanks to Catherine Wire Roberts, who has now edited four books for us. She is not only talented, but her precision to detail and help with bringing each project together with ease never ceases to amaze me. With her full-time job and family commitments, I am forever grateful to her for making time for us, since she provides not only a clarity, but a special touch on each of our books.

Finally, I want to thank my partner Jeffrey Batchelor, who came up with the idea for this book. He is responsible for the pictures and design ideas. Not only is he willing to edit, strategize and organize all our books and projects, but he always has my back and that is something that is beyond priceless.

Susan B. Dopart, MS, RD, CDE

Introduction

Over the past several months you have not felt like your usual self. You've been sluggish most of the time, have no get-up-and-go and a sense that something is not quite right. You hoped it would pass, since you've been under a fair amount of stress and sleep has been challenging.

You finally succumb to going to the doctor, thinking you'll be told to lower your stress. The doctor decides to do some blood work, and when the phone rings a few days later, you hear those three dreaded words: "You have diabetes."

What does that mean? How did this happen? I'm too young to have this!

Research suggests that 1 out of 3 adults has pre-diabetes; of this group, 9 out of 10 people don't know that they have pre-diabetes.

A diabetes diagnosis can sneak up on you like an accident, or can slowly develop over many years. It can depend on the type of diabetes and your genetics.

Controlling blood glucose values for diabetes of any kind, type I (**T1**), type 2 (**T2**), gestational (**GDM**), latent autoimmune diabetes in adults (**LADA**), or a maturity onset diabetes of the young (**MODY**), can be more than challenging given all the factors of good blood glucose control.

T1 diabetes, formerly known as juvenile onset, occurs when the pancreas stops all insulin production and requires daily insulin administration. Whether genetics, a virus, or a combination of factors – what causes T1 diabetes is not definitively known. It was once thought that only children get diagnosed with T1 diabetes, but individuals at any age can develop T1. Often older patients with T1 are frequently misdiagnosed with T2 diabetes.

T2 diabetes, formerly known as adult-onset diabetes, is normally characterized by insulin resistance in which the tissues of the body have less insulin sensitivity. It can be genetic and/or brought on by lifestyle. It is now called T2 diabetes since children as young as three years old have been diagnosed, which speaks to the reality of our sedentary lifestyle and highly processed carbohydrate diet. In addition, when a baby is exposed to high glucose levels in utero, its young pancreas has to overwork before birth, which highly increases the likelihood of developing insulin resistance, weight issues and T2 diabetes early in life.

Sometimes a diagnosis of diabetes can be neither T1 nor T2 and can be challenging to diagnose. Other types of diabetes known as LADA or MODY are discussed in the glossary.

Gestational diabetes (GDM) occurs during pregnancy at around 24-28 weeks gestation when the hormones made by the placenta begin to partially block the action of insulin. Women with GDM can be managed with lifestyle changes, oral medications or insulin.

Metabolism starts with conception, showing the influence of our diets on future generations.

———

Growing up with a dad with T2 diabetes, having multiple relatives with diabetes, and being insulin resistant myself, I've devoted my practice and life to learning how to navigate the diabetes world. There's always something new to learn, and I thank my patients for sharing their journeys and struggles with me.

It's never too early to change your lifestyle to improve blood glucose control. Researchers even indicate that a healthy lifestyle for a pregnant woman is essential to preventing her baby from becoming diabetic later in life.

A small change in lifestyle can mean larger shifts in your metabolic system, leading to positive glucose and health changes.

Some of the tips in this book are helpful for some types of diabetes and not for others. I am not differentiating between them for simplicity's sake, but take what you like and leave the rest.

Even if you do not have a diabetes diagnosis, the following information can prevent diabetes in those who are insulin resistant or just wanting to achieve a healthful lifestyle.

Many points are supported by research studies and some are observations from my 25 years of working with those who are insulin resistant and diabetic.

MYTH: If I have diabetes I will know it.

FACT: You can have diabetes for many years without knowing it. Anne Peters, MD, a leading diabetologist and researcher at University of Southern California (USC), believes that the average person diagnosed with T2 diabetes actually had it for seven years prior to diagnosis!

I've divided each section into categories for ease. Some points are linked to studies, some to blogs, and others even to recipes or videos for fun and practicality, so enjoy the quick read.

Share these points with your family members, friends and carry them with you as a fast reference guide. Start living your life in the zone of knowledge and understanding of diabetes prevention and control.

Although diabetes is serious, especially if ignored, it can be a blessing in creating greater awareness about the need to balance your food, be active and maintain a healthy lifestyle. These things are all helpful in avoiding other types of illness and giving you control over how you live your life, what I collectively call your **Recipe for Life**.

SUSAN'S STORY

I remember even at eight years old feeling my clothes were too tight. I knew most of my friends were smaller than me, and that I was ALWAYS HUNGRY.

If I had a Ding Dong after school, I wanted another one. In pursuit of sweets, I continually wanted to make cookies. My mother finally got me my own baking book in second grade so I could make cookies myself, and eventually I became the family baker. I could bake amazing cookies, cakes and treats from scratch without effort.

When I got to college and took my first nutrition class, I realized I wanted to pursue food beyond baking. Having had some health issues in the past, I resolved not to become diabetic and continually struggle with my weight. This started my pursuit of eating well and being healthy. This book is not only a compilation of the current research that exists on health for diabetes, but also includes pointers that have worked for me and my patients.

SBD

Diet and Meal Balance

BREAKFAST AND MORNING ROUTINE

1. Eat breakfast every day. Starting your day with breakfast is one of the best ways to set the tone for blood glucose control. Waiting to eat is a set-up for being over hungry at the next meal, resulting in higher blood glucose levels and playing catch up with your diabetes. Studies show there is a correlation between skipping breakfast and poor glycemic control in T2 diabetes. Those who ate breakfast had a better glycosylated hemoglobin A1C. Even if your fasting glucose level is elevated, it is still important to eat breakfast to assist with improved blood glucose regulation for the remainder of the day.

> "All happiness depends on a leisurely breakfast."
> - John Gunther

2. Eat within 60 minutes of waking. For decades we've been told the importance of breakfast. Still, many think of breakfast as optional, but here are some good reasons to include this important meal on a daily basis.

Eating upon waking contributes to a stronger metabolism, which means you will be more likely to utilize the food you've eaten all throughout the day. Because you are fasting overnight, waiting several hours can lower your metabolism and increase carbohydrate cravings (since your brain needs fuel), which can lead to overeating at other meals later in the day. Eating more of your food later in the day can lead to weight gain and higher blood glucose values.

3. Add protein to breakfast. Protein is one of the keys to controlling blood glucose values. It helps with lowering the spike in insulin caused by carbohydrate alone, and stabilizing the blood glucose curve. Protein helps you feel full, and extends the time till you are hungry again. Research shows breakfast highly influences the A1C. Adding eggs, Greek yogurt, cottage cheese and nut butters to your morning can go a long way toward glycemic control.

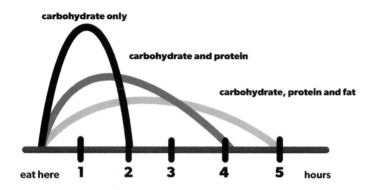

carbohydrate only

carbohydrate and protein

carbohydrate, protein and fat

eat here **1 2 3 4 5** hours

MEAL BALANCE

If you eat a high-carbohydrate, low-protein breakfast, insulin
levels can increase sharply, causing your blood sugar to crash
within 2-2½ hours, stimulating hunger. If you eat a balance of
protein, healthy fat, and moderate amounts of carbohydrate,
insulin levels will rise more moderately, causing your blood
sugars and appetite to be at a more even keel.

4. Keep your carbohydrates low at breakfast. The cells of
your body use insulin less effectively in the morning because you
are just getting up from sleep. As the day progresses, your cells are
more responsive and sensitive to insulin and can effectively handle
a larger amount of carbohydrate. Vegetable carbohydrates and
those contained in fat such as nuts and avocados will fare better
on morning blood glucose values, so skip the bagel and juice.

5. Skip the cereal at breakfast. Eating cereal is like having
a candy bar for breakfast. Cereal contains anywhere from 30-80
grams of carbohydrate per serving, or 2-5 slices worth of bread.
This carbohydrate load can quickly spike your blood glucose readings, creating a high glucose and then a rebound low leading
to more carbohydrate cravings for the remainder of the day.

I ate cereal for breakfast for years, thinking it was a healthy option. Unfortunately I was always starving two hours later. I did not know the connection between eating a high-carb breakfast and increased hunger. If I had, I would have abandoned it years before I did.

SBD

LUNCH/DINNER/MEALS

6. Increase protein and healthy fats at all meals and snacks and lower carbohydrates if you want to create stability in your blood glucose readings. With T2 diabetes there is a "carbohydrate intolerance," so lowering your total carbs and focusing your meals on a higher percentage of protein and good fats can lead to better blood glucose control.

"Diabetes taught me discipline."
- Sonia Sotomayor

---

7. Ensure you have a protein source in every meal.
A protein source will balance your meal and keep your blood glucose values stable and assist with satiation. If you are consuming a veggie burger, add an egg, a slice of cheese or some Greek yogurt. If you are vegan, consider adding more nuts/seeds, nut butter or hummus.

8. Avoid eating after dinner and work at having a 10-12 hour fast overnight, which allows your body to normalize blood glucose levels. For insulin to do its job and reset your metabolism for the next day, it needs to operate in the fasting state. Late dinners and snacks are associated with poor glycemic control in T2 diabetes. Going 12 hours without food can make your cells more sensitive to insulin and metabolize glucose more effectively, which allows your system to reset for another day.

———

I grew up as part of the low-fat, high-carb craze. Not knowing my body needed more protein than most, I lived my college life tired, hungry and iron deficient. It was only when I was educated on insulin resistance and diabetes that weight, hunger and fatigue became a thing of the past.

SBD

———

9. Drink tea with your meals. The polyphenols or antioxidants in tea (green, black or oolong) can lower post meal blood glucose and avoid hyperglycemia. Research links drinking tea with longevity. Tea increases the length of telomeres, DNA complexes on the ends of chromosomes, which are tied to aging.

SNACKS

10. Eat unsalted raw or dry roasted tree nuts, peanuts or seeds for snacks along with carrots, which have a low glycemic index and hardly raise your glucose levels. The glycemic index is a scale from 0-100 with potatoes and white rice near the top with approximate values of 75-90, while most nuts have a glycemic index of 14-20. Although many think carrots are off limits due to a higher glycemic index than other vegetables, the amount is so small on the scale that one would have to consume many carrots to have a high glucose load, making it absurd to not eat carrots.

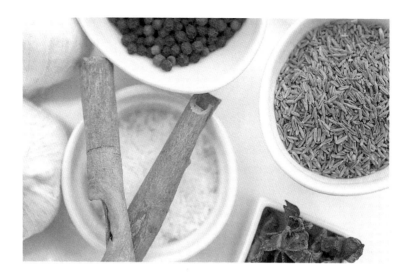

I now substitute dark chocolate for my cookie cravings. I was a former milk chocolate lover. I started with a slightly higher percentage (55 percent to help acclimate to less sweetness) and gradually built up to 85 percent. Brands vary dramatically in taste, but finding one you like is a fun endeavor and can really help out when you need a little treat.

SBD

11. During the day, don't go more than four hours without food. Eating regular meals is essential to keeping glucose values stable, while irregular eating patterns are a set-up for blood glucose highs and lows. If you're eating lunch at noon and dinner at 7 p.m., have a snack around 4 p.m. It will help your energy and prevent the possibility of overeating at dinner.

12. Consuming two squares (about ½ ounce) of high quality dark chocolate (over 75 percent cocoa) is a great way to help your sweet tooth. This snack contains no flour, a limited amount of sugar with cocoa butter, and will hardly raise your glucose levels. Dark chocolate contains polyphenols, which can help insulin sensitivity and artery health. Combine with 1-2 tablespoons of natural peanut or other nut butter and make your own healthy peanut butter cup.

Early diagnosis and treatment of T2 diabetes can be done through relatively inexpensive blood testing.

———

CARBOHYDRATES

Carbohydrates are one of the three macronutrients of which food is comprised. Healthy sources of carbohydrate-containing foods include whole plant foods such as vegetables, fruits, nuts, seeds, beans, legumes and unrefined grains such as brown rice, quinoa — or in essence, those without a label.

Refined sources of carbohydrate include foods you typically find in a package, such as cookies, crackers, cereals, candy, chips, etc.

Choosing carbohydrates in their raw, unprocessed form without a label means you are consuming more fiber. However, matching the carbohydrates you are consuming with your level of insulin resistance, blood glucose values and insulin requirements (if applicable) is still essential, even if you are choosing healthy carbohydrate sources.

13. Keep your carbohydrate level to less than 100 total grams per day. Amounts of carbohydrates needed per day are individual, especially with respect to the type of diabetes. However, for those with insulin resistance and T2, limiting carbohydrate intake per day or per meal can be helpful for good glycemic control and weight loss. Carbohydrate counting can be quite useful for keeping track of your carb intake and helps with being conscious of how many carbs you are actually consuming, empowering your choices for blood glucose control.

MYTH: Now that I have diabetes I can never eat a dessert.

FACT: Managing your blood sugars and diabetes means you have a balance of enough protein, moderate amounts of carbohydrate and good fat at your meals and snacks. Small amounts of sugar, like in dark chocolate, have minimal effect on your glucose levels if consumed in moderate quantities.

14. Keep your carbohydrates under 25 grams within a four hour period. This recommendation is quite individual and mostly applies to T2s. Those with T2 diabetes generally have a "carbohydrate intolerance." Restricting carbohydrates, especially within a timeframe, allows the pancreas to "rest" and your body to process the carbohydrates you are consuming. Not overloading your pancreas with a high carbohydrate intake decreases its stress, allowing it to rest. Your pancreas responds to excessive intake of carbohydrate by secreting more insulin, which can result in rebound hypoglycemia. This signals your body to crave more food, particularly carbohydrate. Consuming excess carbs can start a cycle of hunger, which signals the body to want more carbohydrates, resulting in a physiologic pattern of poor food choices.

15. Consume less than 50 grams of total carbohydrate per day if your glycosylated A1C is above 8.0 mg/dl. Consuming fewer carbohydrates can lower insulin resistance and result in a reduction in the A1C.

16. Eat your carbohydrates from non-starch sources.
Consuming carbohydrates from veggies, nuts/seeds, plain dairy products and minimal fruit can be helpful for lowering glucose values. Although fruit is healthy, over-consuming fruit can quickly

tip you over your carbohydrate allotment. Eating fruit paired with a healthy fat or protein slows the absorption of carbohydrate in the bloodstream. By slowing the impact of glucose, your body has more time to metabolize the glucose, thereby decreasing its impact.

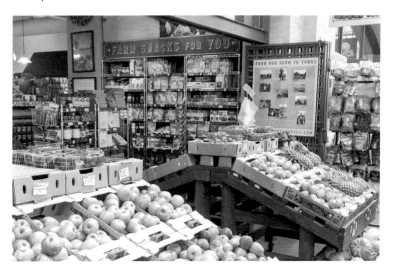

17. Avoid processed carbohydrates. Consuming packaged cookies, chips and other processed "foods" is a set-up for high glucose readings. They contain large amounts of sugar, high fructose corn syrup, trans fat and other additives. Shopping around the periphery of the grocery store can help keep you safe from processed carb temptation.

18. Limit even "healthy" whole grains or starches, since they can increase blood glucose readings. One way to assess how whole grains, brown rice, quinoa or potatoes impact your blood glucose is to test your values one and half hours after the first bite of a meal. One cup of healthy brown rice contains 45 grams of carbohydrate or three slices of bread, which may be more carbohydrate than someone with T2 can handle at one time. Being mindful of your serving size of starches is essential to achieving good blood glucose control.

19. Match your morning "report card" with your carbohydrate intake. How do you figure this out? If you are a T2, your morning blood sugar is the report card to let you know if you overshot your carbohydrate consumption the previous day. Throughout the day, carbohydrate that is not utilized by your body can be stored as fat or get shuttled to the liver. Overnight your liver can release the extra glucose into your bloodstream, which will result in a higher morning blood glucose level than when you went to bed. This additional glucose storage in the liver is a setup for nonalcoholic fatty liver disease.

MYTH: Since I now have a diagnosis of diabetes, it feels like a death sentence.

FACT: Type 2 diabetes is extremely controllable with lifestyle and medications. It is not a death sentence by any stretch, and if managed daily, can keep your life in balance.

20. Decide how you want to spend your carbohydrate allotment for the day. Which carbs are the most important to you (ones you will miss if you don't include them) and which types of carbs are not that essential to your lifestyle? A slice of bread at dinner may mean skipping the fruit or "exchanging" it for another type of carbohydrate so you don't exceed your daily allotment.

21. Look at "total carbs" on a label rather than "sugar," since total carbohydrates include the sugar. Approximately 15 grams of carbohydrate is equal to one slice of bread. A regular-sized bagel contains 60 grams of total carbs or four slices worth of bread. Since we live in a carb society, your carb intake can add up quickly leading to higher blood glucose values.

22. Limit high carb meals, since just one can increase insulin resistance and lower fat metabolism for up to seven days. Consuming more carbohydrates than your body can handle for even one meal a day or a week can sabotage weight loss and lead to higher glucose levels throughout the week. Ask yourself, "Is this one meal worth higher blood glucose values for the entire week?"

23. Be aware there is a spectrum of insulin resistance among individuals. When someone with normal insulin sensitivity consumes a slice of bread, their body secretes enough insulin to allow that slice to be metabolized. In the body of someone with a high level of insulin resistance, however, their body could respond as if it had nine slices. Research shows those with the most insulin resistance can have nine times the normal hyperinsulinemic response to food – meaning the body secretes nine times more insulin than normal when consuming a slice of bread, which can quickly increase weight/fat gain, cravings and hunger levels.

———

Being Italian and insulin resistant was challenging for family dinners. However, I have found substitutes that satisfy, such as squash for pasta, cauliflower for potatoes, and Portobello mushrooms for pizza. These are well worth the payoff of less hunger, lower glucose levels and more energy.

SBD

———

24. Match carbohydrate with proteins to help with blood glucose stabilization and satiation. So, if you are eating an apple, add a slice or two of cheese or an ounce of nuts.

CARBOHYDRATE SUBSTITUTES

25. Use Portobello mushrooms for a crust, when making a pizza. Scoop out the mushroom insides and bake 5-10 minutes, which will lower the moisture in the mushrooms. Then add tomato sauce or paste, cheese, and other toppings and broil for a few minutes until desired doneness. Many recipes also exist for tasty crusts made with cauliflower, although they require more effort than using mushrooms.

26. Substitute zucchini or eggplant for noodles in lasagna. Layer the vegetable just as you would the pasta and top with tomato sauce, ricotta cheese, mozzarella cheese and ground turkey or beef, as desired. It is quite tasty, provides a vegetable serving or two and will save you 20-40 grams of carbohydrates per serving.

27. Substitute cauliflower for potatoes. Make mashed cauliflower or cauliflower au gratin or twice-baked cauliflower. Roast the cauliflower with garlic and add milk, butter, cheese or sour cream in a blender or food processor. If making twice baked, put mixture in ramekins and top with white cheddar cheese and bake until hot and bubbly. You will save 20-25 grams of carbohydrates per cup serving besides increasing nutrients.

Making substitutes for food high in starch can lower insulin resistance, leading to decreased glucose values and reducing the amount of medication and/or insulin needed.

────

28. Swap out spaghetti squash for pasta. You'll lower your carbs and increase nutrients simultaneously.

29. Eat pasta al dente if you must fulfill your pasta craving. The pasta will have less effect on increasing your blood glucose readings due to having a lower glycemic index and higher amounts of resistant starch.

REGULAR METABOLISM OF CARBOHYDRATE

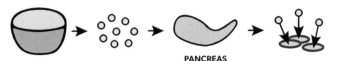

	PANCREAS	
digested in the body	broken down to sugar/glucose which needs to enter the cells	sugar/glucose enter the cells

The pancreas produces insulin, which is the key that unlocks the cells for sugar/glucose to enter.

INSULIN RESISTANCE
there are three possible scenarios

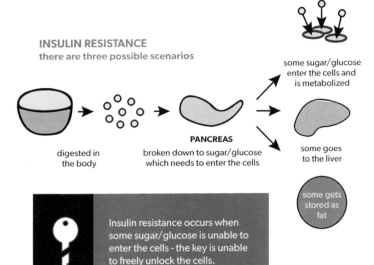

some sugar/glucose enter the cells and is metabolized

some goes to the liver

some gets stored as fat

digested in the body

PANCREAS
broken down to sugar/glucose which needs to enter the cells

Insulin resistance occurs when some sugar/glucose is unable to enter the cells - the key is unable to freely unlock the cells.

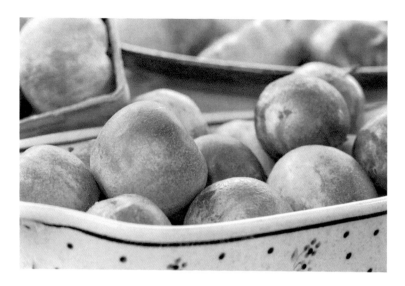

FRUIT

30. Limit your intake of fruit. Although fruit is a healthy carbohydrate with fiber included, it can increase your glucose values if consumed in significant portions. Limit portions to ½ cup, one medium, or ½ large fruit and consume as your blood glucose values allow in your carbohydrate allotment. In general, berries have less carbs than other types of fruit.

31. Make sure the bananas you're consuming are a touch under-ripe. Eating bananas with a touch of green means they have more "resistant starch," which can improve digestion and absorption, thereby not raising blood glucose values as much as a ripened or spotted banana. One study showed that resistant starch improved first phase insulin secretion in T2 diabetes. Avoid riper bananas with spots.

32. Limit your intake of grapes and cherries. Depending on their size, grapes and cherries contain between ½-1 gram of carbohydrate each. Eating just one cup can mean you are consuming as much as 30 grams of carbohydrate, or two slices worth of bread. Mindfulness is key since eating an entire bowl of grapes is easy to do, similar to eating a bowl of popcorn.

BEVERAGES

33. Avoid beverages with carbohydrates. Whether it is soda, juice or a sweetened beverage, drinking beverages with carbohydrates is a quick way to spike glucose values, which usually results in a drop later, creating a yo-yo effect in glucose values.

34. Make sure to look at how many "servings" are contained in the beverage you are drinking. The carbohydrate label amount may be only 5-10 grams, but containers of beverages can contain two servings per container, so you may be taking in more carbs than you realize.

───────

I used to love my mocha lattes a few days a week. However, when I learned the carb content, I switched to tea and coffee. If I want a little treat, I add cinnamon, a shake of cocoa and some half and half to my café.

SBD

───────

35. Drink iced tea or sparkling water with lemon or natural flavoring. Avoid diet drinks, lemonade or sodas to control carbohydrate intake. Consider adding sparkling water to iced tea for a different twist.

36. Avoid specialty coffee drinks. They can contain large amounts of carbohydrate/sugar. One coffee drink can contain 45-90 grams of carbohydrate in just one beverage! If you're not careful, you could be drinking a "loaf" of bread.

37. To sweeten coffee, use unsweetened cocoa powder and cinnamon and avoid the sugar, sweeteners, etc. Avoiding the flavored creamers can save you a slice of bread's worth of carbohydrate.

I used to have a diet soda most afternoons around 3 p.m. Twenty years ago, after drinking one, my blood sugar dropped dramatically. I became nauseous, was shaking and had to delay my next patient. I thought nothing of it until the next day when it happened again within 10 minutes of drinking my 3 p.m. diet soda. I realized the connection between artificial sweeteners and hypoglycemia, and therefore have not had one since.

SBD

38. Make your tea more interesting by adding fresh squeezed lemon or a ½ teaspoon of raw honey. Raw honey has good probiotics and natural sweetness, versus fake sweeteners or sugar.

39. Limit your consumption of alcohol. Alcohol breaks down into sugar and is stored by the liver, which is a set-up for creating instability in your readings. Some experience a drop followed by a rise in glucose readings following alcohol consumption. So, if you imbibe, make sure to know how alcohol affects your system. In addition, drinking lowers your inhibition, which can set you up for overeating. Being tempted by the fancy drink list or signature cocktails may lead you down a road that is not celebratory over the rest of your week. If you want an adult beverage, consider sticking with a shot of vodka or small glass of wine.

40. Limit your consumption of caffeine from coffee. Caffeine from coffee can increase insulin levels by 42 percent and decrease insulin sensitivity by 25 percent since it increases stress levels in the body, thereby raising blood glucose levels. In addition, coffee has the ability to induce hypoglycemia.

Adding to Your Meals

CONDIMENTS AND FOOD ADDITIVES

41. Watch your condiments! Every tablespoon of the average ketchup or barbeque sauce can contain significant carbs. Just 2 tablespoons of ketchup contains eight carbs or ½ slice of bread. Two tablespoons of barbeque sauce can contain 15-20 grams. Salad dressing can also contain significant amounts of carbohydrates, especially if it is "fat-free," which translates to more carbohydrates.

My whole family loves ketchup. Ketchup was a normal part of consuming hamburgers and eggs, among other foods. This one was a slow wean. I changed to un-sweetened ketchup and eventually got my taste buds on board for using mustard on my food for less carbs and no sugar.

SBD

---

42. Beware of sweeteners that say "low glycemic index."
Agave is touted as great for diabetes, but it is 85 percent fructose, or double the fructose of high fructose corn syrup (HFCS). Fructose that is extracted as a syrup goes straight to the liver and can increase both weight gain and fatty liver.

43. Avoid non-nutritive sweeteners. In addition to increasing your threshold for wanting sweet, research shows diet drinks and foods can make your body secrete more insulin, which can cause weight gain, increased cravings, and fluctuation in blood glucose values. Recent studies showed they even change your gut hormones, which can increase weight gain.

44. Use dill pickled relish, rather than sweet relish. Sweet relish contains sugar or high fructose corn syrup, so you could be adding a slice of bread's worth of carbs to your tuna salad.

"Fat is not the problem. If Americans could eliminate sugary beverages, potatoes, white bread, pasta, white rice and sugary snacks, we would wipe out almost all the problems we have with weight and diabetes and other metabolic diseases."
- Walter Willett, MD,
Harvard School of Public Health

———

45. Watch the amount of tomato or spaghetti sauce you consume. Although tomatoes are healthy, tomato or spaghetti sauce can contain more carbohydrates than your body can handle, as some have added sugar. One cup can contain between 12-30 grams of carbohydrates. Consuming 2 cups on top of your already high carbohydrate pasta can quickly spike your readings. Consider making your own homemade recipe from fresh tomatoes with no sugar added.

46. Use a good quality extra-virgin olive oil for low temperature cooking (200-400°F) and in dressings and marinades. Olive oil is a healthy monounsaturated fat that contains many health-promoting properties such as polyphenols, which are powerful antioxidants. Studies show olive oil protects the endothelium or lining of your blood vessels, which can be compromised with diabetes. Using olive oil in high temperature cooking is thought to damage the antioxidants as well as the taste. Recommended oils for high temperature cooking are grapeseed oil and extra-virgin organic coconut oil.

47. Spice it up! Studies show that highly spiced foods can lower your appetite and give you that satisfied or full feeling, which can lead to less food intake and lower blood glucose values. Curry powder, turmeric, and pepper are some examples.

FOOD EXTRAS

48. Avoid "instant" products like instant oatmeal or packaged foods that contain large amounts of carbohydrates and are quite low in fiber, a good combination to increase blood glucose. In addition, a high glycemic carbohydrate diet has been linked with high insulin levels, which is related to incidences of cancer.

49. Add avocado to meals to increase satiation. Studies show that avocados increased satiety following a meal by 26 percent and decreased the desire to eat by 40 percent, which may be due to both its fat and fiber content. Just one half of an avocado contains 7 grams of fiber, as well as healthy monounsaturated fat to help with lowering constipation and increasing gut motility.

50. Eat nut butter for dessert. Consuming natural peanut, almond or cashew butter with carrots or celery can satisfy a sweet craving without raising blood glucose values significantly. To make your own, combine peanuts and cashews with avocado oil and a touch of sea salt and blend in food processor for a decadent treat!

The fat-free era, which vilified fat, resulted in a plethora of fat-free products, which gave the false illusion of health and healthy food options.

——

51. Avoid imitation crabmeat. Although real crabmeat contains no carbohydrate, the imitation kind contains approximately 15 grams per half cup serving due to added wheat starch and sweeteners.

52. Avoid fat-free products. They are generally full of sugar. For example, a fat-free salad dressing can contain corn syrup, sugar, and other sweeteners for as much as 15 grams of carbohydrate for just 2 tablespoons.

53. Beware of veggie burgers, which can be made of corn, rice, beans and other carbohydrate-containing foods. Veggie burgers range from 10-40 grams of carbohydrate per patty, so check the labels or ask your server what ingredients it contains.

54. Increase all forms of fiber, especially vegetables, nuts/seeds, chia and ground flax seeds. Fiber lowers blood glucose values by slowing gastric emptying and carbohydrate absorption. Increase fiber intake over time to allow the stomach to acclimate to the diet change.

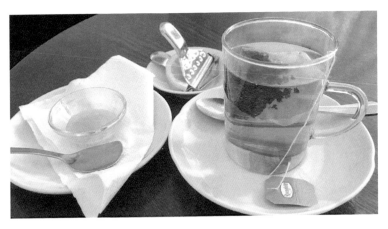

55. Consider adding foods high in polyphenols to your diet. Studies show a diet high in polyphenols lowers glucose values and increases sensitivity to the early phase of insulin secretion. Foods that contain polyphenols include berries, apples, tea and ground flax seeds. Adding berries to plain yogurt topped with sliced almonds makes for a nice breakfast or snack.

56. Add choline-rich foods to your diet. Choline is essential for the brain. It's also associated with low incidence of fatty liver. The recommended intake of choline per day is 250 mg. Since a single egg yolk contains 125 mg., consuming two eggs per day meets your choline requirements in addition to containing the optimal amino acid profile of any food to help stabilize blood glucose values. Although eggs were once considered taboo due to their high cholesterol content, research indicates that the link between egg consumption and cholesterol values was based on out-of-date information.

57. Add a food high in probiotics or a supplement. Since diabetes is tied to gut hormones, maintaining a healthy gut is essential to favorable blood glucose values. Foods high in natural probiotics include plain yogurt, kefir, and fermented foods such as sauerkraut, also known as a cultured vegetable. If you cannot tolerate these foods, consider a supplement. When selecting a probiotic, consider one with at least 25 billion CFUs (colon-forming units). CFUs represent the ability of the bacteria to survive acidity of the stomach. Some probiotics need refrigeration, since they are live bacteria that need to be maintained in a cold environment, which also increases their shelf life. Other manufacturers claim their probiotics are freeze-dried and don't require refrigeration.

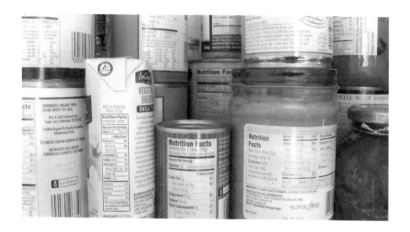

LABELS

58. Read labels and limit foods that have more than 5-6 ingredients. Foods that contain multiple ingredients are more processed, which usually means higher levels of carbohydrates.

59. Consume more foods that don't require a label, such as vegetables, salads, fruit, etc. Nature's food contains more fiber, which means lower blood glucose readings. Shopping on the perimeter of the grocery store and more often at farmers' markets, can help transition your lifestyle to healthier high fiber foods.

At the height of my sugar cravings, I would frequently visit a Chinese restaurant and order Orange Chicken. Little did I know I was eating three slices worth of bread in my order with only two ounces of protein, since it contains mostly sugar and starch.

SBD

EATING OUT: WHAT IS BEHIND THAT MENU?

60. Be wary of Chinese food. Even if you avoid the white rice and noodles, the sauces in Chinese food contain sugars and cornstarch, which can add up to a fair amount of carbohydrates, driving up glucose levels. If you are consuming Chinese food, stick to beef and broccoli, chicken and vegetables and avoid sweet and sour, lemon and orange sauces.

61. Be wary of Mexican food, which also contains high amounts of carbohydrates. Eat the fajitas with one corn tortilla or ½ cup beans, which is equal to approximately 15-20 grams of carbohydrate. Starches abound in Mexican food. The rice, beans, tortillas, and chips can add up significant levels of carbohydrates, without even counting the Margaritas. Choose the carbs that are the most important to your meal.

62. Don't be fooled by a "healthy" sushi meal, which can be high in carbohydrates. One sushi roll can contain as much as 45-60 grams of total carbohydrates, or 3-4 slices worth of bread. Sushi rice is high in starches and contains added sugar to increase the stickiness. Stick to the sashimi, Yakitori sticks, vegetables, salad and miso soup.

63. Watch the teriyaki sauce when eating Japanese food as it is high in carbohydrate, and you could be eating a carbohydrate serving of bread in just the sauce on your chicken. One tablespoon contains between 4-8 grams of carbohydrate, and since the amount added to an entrée could easily be 4-6 tablespoons, 15-50 grams of carbohydrate will be added to your meal.

"29.1 million people in the United States have diabetes, 8.1 million of whom may be undiagnosed and unaware of their condition." Centers for Disease Control and Prevention (CDC)

——

MYTH: If you are thin you are not at risk for diabetes.

FACT: One can be diagnosed with diabetes regardless of body type.

64. Don't put your pancreas into a 911 state. The weekend is a time for relaxing and enjoyment, but excess carbohydrates can sabotage the rest your pancreas needs for the weekend. Since the blood stream can only process approximately 8-10 grams of carbohydrates within a short timeframe, consuming a sweetened coffee drink and a bagel can contain as much as 150 grams of carbohydrate. Limiting your carbohydrates to very small amounts throughout the day allows your liver and pancreas to "rest" thus controlling both your blood sugar and weight! How's that for a win-win?

Extras

ACTIVITY AND EXERCISE

65. Exercise or be active for 10 minutes after every meal. Exercising or activity after a meal makes your insulin 30-40 percent more sensitive, and drives the food you just consumed into your cells. A study of women who had GDM showed that more than half of the women lowered their blood glucose values without the need for insulin 10 days after initiating an exercise program.

If I had my preference, I would work out in the afternoon, but that doesn't fit my lifestyle. I consider going to the gym or morning exercise like brushing my teeth – it's mandatory if I want to lower my insulin resistance and maintain my weight. I set out my gym clothes before bed and get up at the crack of dawn so I'm done before work.

SBD

---

66. Exercise for 30 minutes a day. Exercise is like a magic pill to help control glucose values. The muscles in your body contain a compound known as glut4, which is activated during exercise. This compound allows glucose to get into the cells with less insulin. In addition, exercise is associated with lowered risk of Alzheimer's, cardiovascular disease and cancer.

67. Have a walk for dessert. Researchers found that those with T1 diabetes who took a walk after a meal had 145 percent lower blood glucose values than those who didn't walk for as long as 4½ hours following the meal.

68. Get up and move at least once every 30-60 minutes. Moving as much as possible allows your insulin receptors to be more sensitive to the glucose that is trying to get into your cells. Sitting time really does matter and contributes to higher glucose values. Little extras such as a quick vacuum, a dusting around the house, or walking upstairs to put something away can all add up and go a long way toward blood glucose control. If you're watching TV in the evenings, stand up during commercial breaks to utilize the benefits of glut4 (which helps with lowering glucose so less insulin is needed).

69. Get your glucose values down by taking a 20-minute walk and/or consuming a mostly protein-based meal with non-starchy vegetables at your next meal. Just one walk can increase your insulin sensitivity for a few days. Retest your values after the walk and see how significant one walk can be. However, if your blood glucose is higher than 250 mg/dl, refrain from exercise as this may cause your values to go higher. In that case, recommendations are for gentle walking until your glucose values are lower.

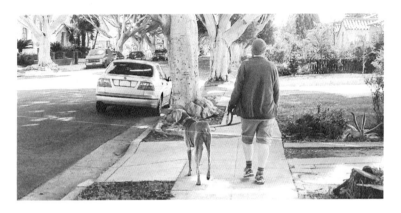

"I do not love to work out, but if I stick to exercising every day and put the right things in my mouth, then my diabetes stays in check."
- Halle Berry

70. Get a pedometer or device to count your activity and steps. Accumulating 10,000 steps per day is associated with lowering insulin resistance and glucose values. Consider ways to move more such as gardening, vacuuming, or washing your car.

71. Exercise in the morning. Since you are the most insulin resistant early in the day, exercise and/or activity increase insulin sensitivity for the remainder of the day.

72. Walk the dog. They will become more fit and you'll make your insulin more sensitive.

73. Consider ways to sit less since sitting is the new smoking. Try walking to deliver a message to co-workers versus sending an email, standing while on a phone call or walking to lunch or dinner a few days of the week. These small changes can go a long way toward helping lower glucose values by lowering insulin resistance.

> Large population studies show that
> 8,000-12,000 steps per day are associated
> with better health outcomes.

LIFESTYLE

74. Take a happiness break each day. During that break, do something that makes you truly happy. Happiness produces endorphins, which can lower stress in the body, leading to lower blood glucose values. High stress is associated with higher blood glucose values. If you are at a high stress job, smile and imagine a better place for a moment, which may go a long way toward lowering your stress and glucose levels.

75. Don't stress about high blood glucose values, but do avoid stress foods. Since knowledge is power, observe when your blood glucose goes up or down so you can problem-solve for the next time. Getting stressed out increases your cortisol levels (the stress hormone) in your body, which can, in turn, push blood glucose higher. Avoiding stress foods (sugary processed foods) can go a long way toward better blood glucose control. Practice stress-reducing techniques everyday, such as breathing and mindfulness, so when stressful situations come up you are prepared.

76. Take a few little 1-2 minute stress breaks during the day, so you can process your thoughts. Increased stress in your body can build throughout the day, leading to higher blood sugars, thus increasing carb cravings, which lead to stress eating.

77. Spend more time in the kitchen. Research shows those who cook at home eat more healthfully, besides saving money and time.

MYTH: Now that I have diabetes I'm afraid I will go blind or have an amputation.

FACT: Controlling your blood sugars means having little to no risk of health issues such as eye disease or having to undergo amputations. A blood test known as *glycosylated hemoglobin A1C* shows what your blood glucose values are averaging over a three-month period. Keeping that number in range dramatically lowers the risk of medical complications.

78. Review your prescription drugs with your doctor and pharmacist. Various classifications of drugs, including those for blood pressure, birth control and psychotropic drugs, have the potential of increasing insulin resistance leading to higher glucose values and weight gain.

79. Keep a food diary. Research shows that just the habit of writing down your food consumption increases self-awareness and weight loss. Food diaries can also work well with correlating food and blood glucose values.

80. Avoid the break room or places in your work environment that trigger overeating. Break rooms are generally places especially prone to easy sources of sugary, starchy carbs. Environmental control can be key to keeping your glucose values in control.

81. Consider the use of an app if you need to be more aware of how many carbohydrates you are taking in or your diet balance.

82. Be aware of "diabetes distress." Having a constant medical condition in your body at all times is more than challenging and requires daily management of diet, exercise and sleep. Consider extra support from family, medical and psychological professionals.

When I worked at UCLA, every nursing station was like a continual break room of donuts, cookies, candy and treats from patients' families spoiling the staff. I eventually had to practice self control to not eat anything, or else I would be snacking all day. However, I made sure to have a high protein snack with me at all times to ensure I had an option.

SBD

---

83. Stick to a schedule with your diet, exercise and sleep. Although life can be challenging and changing, diabetes likes consistency, so controlling what you can (meals, exercise, timing of medications) will go a long way toward helping stabilize blood glucose values. The famous DCCT trial (Diabetes Control and Complications Trial) showed lifestyle management was associated with lower all-cause mortality. Diabetes does not take a vacation, so ongoing management is the key to lower glucose values.

84. Lose 10 pounds if your blood glucose values don't seem to be budging. Research shows that a 10-pound weight loss with T2 diabetes can significantly lower blood glucose values and A1C - a two for two win! Weight loss "rests" the beta-cells of your pancreas, which produce insulin so resting them can delay the progression of diabetes, thus delaying the need for more medication and/or insulin. In addition, a 10-pound weight loss can lower blood pressure and decrease pressure on your skeletal system.

85. Organize your food for the week. Taking the time to make a few large entrees to ensure leftovers, such as a roasted chicken, frittata, tuna salad and other protein-rich items, can save you time during the week and ensure you have blood glucose friendly meals on hand, preventing both hypoglycemia and reaching for additional easy-to-find carbohydrates. Planning for meals versus coming up with last minute meals will help with thoughtful food choices, thus avoiding last minute emergencies.

86. Lower your amount of "screen time" such as watching TV, Internet surfing, Facebook and emails. A recent statistic showed people spend 74 minutes per day browsing the Internet and 81 minutes per day using their smartphones for a whopping total of 155 minutes or 2.5 hours per day. Swapping out 15 minutes of screen time per day with an activity can increase glucose disposal by the muscles by activating glut4, which will lower readings.

"Replacing 60 minutes of TV time with a 60-minute stroll would increase a person's chance of living five years longer by 40 percent."
- *Medicine and Science in Sports and Exercise,*
February 2016

___

SLEEP

87. Get at least 7.5 hours of sleep per night. Adequate rest increases the sensitivity of your insulin. Studies continue to show that those getting less than 7.5 hours per night are more insulin resistant. Inadequate sleep results in higher levels of the hormone ghrelin, which grows your appetite, and lower levels of the hormone leptin, which lowers your appetite.

88. Practice good sleep hygiene – and this does not include brushing your eyelids. An hour before bed, turn off all electronics, including the computer, TV, iPads and phones. These devices keep your brain active and awake, which challenges getting to sleep, thereby raising blood glucose values for the next day.

TRAVEL

89. Carefully plan your travel. Plan not only your travel arrangements, but also plan your meals and medication needs. Since diabetes likes consistency, be mindful when crossing time zones and plan for how you will coordinate your meal timing and medication. Research if your airline has meals that are appropriate for you and don't be afraid to ask hotels for assistance. Having a refrigerator in your room for storing snacks, medications and insulin can be helpful.

90. Adequately hydrate on your trip. While being on planes, trains and in automobiles, self-care is extremely important for good blood glucose control. Drinking water or sparkling water for hydration helps with fatigue and headache prevention. The altitude and dry air on airplanes, coupled with alcohol consumption, is not a great combo for diabetes control, so stick to the free movies for entertainment.

> **MYTH:** If your blood glucose levels are elevated, you will feel it in your body.
>
> **FACT:** Diabetes is usually silent until your blood sugars are painfully high. Subtle signs may be having more carbohydrate or sugar cravings, or feeling fatigued or lack of energy even after having a good night's sleep.

SUPPLEMENTS

91. Take vitamin D3. Low levels of vitamin D are associated with both a risk of diabetes and higher mortality. Vitamin D is a hormone and affects over 2,000 systems in the body. It can assist with anything from lowering risk of cancer, to assisting with weight loss, and even avoiding a cold or the flu.

92. Take a fish oil supplement daily or consume wild fish at least 2x/week. Fish and fish oil contain the important omega 3s DHA and EPA, which lower inflammation and triglyceride levels, commonly elevated in those with diabetes. One study showed fatty fish and fish oil may reduce the risk of LADA (latent autoimmune diabetes in adults) as well.

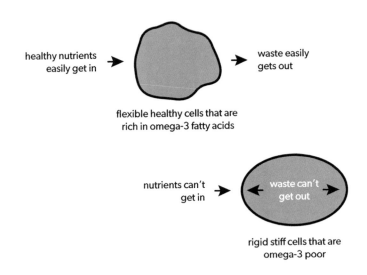

healthy nutrients easily get in → ← waste easily gets out

flexible healthy cells that are
rich in omega-3 fatty acids

nutrients can't get in → ← waste can't get out →

rigid stiff cells that are
omega-3 poor

93. Consume 1-2 tablespoons of ground or milled flax seed on your food per day (yogurt, cottage cheese, salads, etc.). Ground flax seeds provides the third omega 3 ALA that contains a lignin to help not only control blood glucose levels but can also contribute to hormone stabilization. Ground flax seed is thought to be almost like a "Pac-man," gobbling up the harmful hormones in the body to lower risk of cancer and heart disease. For a fantastic review on all the benefits of ground flax seeds see this site: www.whfoods.com/genpage.php?tname=foodspice&dbid=81

94. Take alpha lipoic acid. Alpha lipoic acid is an antioxidant supplement that helps lower blood glucose and can assist with neuropathy pain. Optimal dosage is 600-1,200 mg. per day, depending on symptoms.

95. Take the herb berberine. A few small studies showed that those with T2 diabetes taking 500 mg. three times a day of the herb berberine had a significant decrease in A1C and fasting glucose levels, similar to decreases in those taking Metformin.

96. Use the supplement inositol to lower insulin resistance. Inositol is a naturally occurring vitamin-like substance found in many plants. Since it facilitates serotonin and neurotransmitters in the brain, inositol has been effective in small studies for mood disorders, anxiety and mild depression. It has also been used with metabolic disorders such as insulin resistance, and polycystic ovarian syndrome (PCOS) since it increases insulin sensitivity. Some research suggests it may even be helpful in slowing the progression of diabetic kidney disease. Recommendations vary, so check with your health care provider for dosages.

"Life is not over if you have diabetes.
Make the most of what you have and be grateful."
- Dale Rogers

―――

97. Consider adding N-Acetyl Cysteine (NAC) to your regimen. NAC comes from the amino acid L-cysteine. NAC is effective at lowering insulin resistance, assisting with lung and liver damage and heart health. N-acetyl cysteine has many uses from being an antioxidant to reducing inflammation. Therapeutic levels are from 500 mg. to 3,000 mg. per day.

98. Consider taking the supplement coenzyme Q10 in the form of ubiquinol. Ubiquinol is the reduced form of coenzyme Q10, a naturally occurring antioxidant made in the heart, kidney, liver and pancreas. It is known for fighting free radicals, which are byproducts or spin-offs of normal reactions in the body produced by pollution, smoke or just the normal aging process. Over time, accumulation of free radicals can contribute to heart disease, cancer, weight gain or premature aging, all of which are all associated with diabetes. In addition, many with diabetes take statin drugs and ubiquinol can assist with protection of cell structure and avoiding the aches and pains associated with statin use. Some studies link higher levels of coenzyme Q10 with less chance of diabetic retinopathy.

"You don't have to let your life be destroyed by diabetes. You can reclaim your life."
- Della Reese

___

MEDICATIONS AND INSULIN

99. Give your insulin time to work. If your values are high and you've given yourself extra insulin, don't give yourself more if your values are still high an hour or two later. In doing so, you may be "stacking" your insulin, meaning giving yourself more insulin on top of what is already working, which can lead to hypoglycemia.

100. Monitor your blood glucose levels daily by checking first thing in the morning and at least one other time 1.5-2 hours after the first bite of food. Keeping track of your blood glucose values allows you to see how various food combinations affect your levels. Since each person is sensitive to different types and amounts of carbohydrates, self-monitoring gives you knowledge (which is power) about how specific foods affect your body. Set a timer on your phone for when to test so you don't miss the window of test time.

101. Consider a continuous glucose monitor (CGM) if your blood glucose levels are challenging to control. It might give you insight into your patterns and responses to food, exercise, and stress.

EXTRA TIPS TO CONTROL GLUCOSE VALUES

Take your carb-friendly list to the grocery store. Having a plan for what you are buying and going to make for the week helps with getting in and out of the grocery store without too much carb damage. Make sure you have a snack or meal before your outing to the store, since going hungry is a set-up for buying things you had not intended.

Mind your bites. Mindfulness during meals and snacks goes a long way toward satiation and enjoyment of the food you consume, which decreases chances of overconsumption, leading to better blood glucose control.

Keep your gut healthy. Gut health is a popular health and research topic these days. Your gut is the largest organ in the body after your skin, so what you consume can affect many of your systems. Eating healthful meals that are diabetic-friendly sets the stage for keeping your diabetes and health under control.

Beware of junk foods that are marketed as healthy or good for diabetics. Since diabetes represents a large percentage of the population, food manufacturers spend billions of dollars each year marketing their products as healthful, especially with respect to diabetes. Be aware that there are no "miracle" cures. If it sounds too good to be true, it probably is and best to leave on the shelf.

Consider anti-inflammatory eating. Less inflammation in your system equates to less risk of multiple health issues in the body such as arthritis, cancer, heart disease and diabetes. Choosing your food and its sourcing is essential to diabetes control.

Make your movie experience diabetic-friendly. Although many stay at home and enjoy movies on Netflix, going to see the latest flick in a theater can be a setup for high glucose values. Bringing your own snack or going to the movies right after a meal is better for your blood glucose and your health!

MEDICATIONS FOR DIABETES

Since diabetes is progressive, medication at some point in time may be needed and deemed necessary. Fortunately, there are many options available to help treat diabetes, which was not always the case.

Lifestyle is the first and foremost way to treat T2 diabetes and may be all that is necessary in some cases. In the majority of cases, an oral medication will be needed, and in others insulin is necessary. Your care provider will choose medication based on your particular situation, their own personal experiences with what has worked with their patients, and lists from particular insurance providers.

Discuss with your health care provider your options for medications to help manage your glucose. Share your concerns and challenges and ask them about their experiences with other patients. Be mindful that choices are often made by what your insurance company is willing to pay for. Ask your provider if they have a sample, since trying a medication for a month will help you decide if the product is best for you and agrees with your system.

If your insurance company will not pay for the particular medication your provider prescribes, and you determine it is the best option, there are usually several options in the same class of medications that may be covered.

If all else fails, consider contacting the drug manufacturer or insurance company directly for their assistance.

WHY MEDICATION?

Since high glucose readings are dangerous to the body, medication is a way to allow glucose to enter the cells where it is used for energy. The presence of extra glucose in the body can cause damage to your vascular system.

Many times, medications can be used temporarily while you are adjusting your lifestyle to having diabetes. Some can even support lifestyle management as they promote weight loss. If your glucose is elevated, you may want to consider their use to prevent future complications.

The following list is a summary of some of the most common classifications and names of medications available with a short explanation of how they work and their usefulness in treatment.

In 1942, the first oral type 2 diabetes medication was identified, a sulfonylurea.

———

SULFONYLUREAS

First prescribed in 1955, sulfonylureas stimulate the beta-cells of the pancreas to produce more insulin. Names for sulfonylureas are **Glyburide**, **Glipizide** and **Glimepiride**. They are taken once or twice daily with meals.

Adverse effects are hypoglycemia and weight gain, which are reasons why these medications are not commonly prescribed, and they can compound the problem of weight management with diabetes. In addition, research is leaning towards "resting" the beta-cells of the pancreas so one does not have to go on insulin therapy until needed. Since sulfonylureas drive the beta-cells to produce more insulin, this therapy may not be the best choice unless other options are not desirable for a specific medical concern.

Sulfonylureas are commonly prescribed because they are inexpensive. Many HMOs only have sulfonylureas, Metformin and insulin on their formularies, which is something to be aware of when deciding on which medication works for your needs.

BIGUANIDES

The only medication currently available in this category is **Metformin.** Metformin helps lower the blood glucose by decreasing the amount of glucose production by the liver, thereby increasing your body's response to its own insulin and lowering the amount of glucose from the food you consume. The level of insulin resistance in the body is decreased, which can assist in keeping your glucose levels under control.

Metformin is usually the first medication to be given as it treats the cause of T2: insulin resistance. Metformin is usually taken once or twice a day with meals.

It is not recommended for those with liver or kidney disease, although it's safe for others. Adverse effects may be gastro-intestinal distress, although this can be minimized if taken with food and a low carbohydrate diet is followed. There is a black box warning since it carries a rare risk of lactic acidosis, which occurs in .03 of 1,000 cases. In addition, limiting alcohol is recommended when taking Metformin to avoid this concern.

ALPHA-GLUCOSIDASE INHIBITORS

Alpha-Glucosidase Inhibitors came on the market in 1995. Also known as **Acarbose** and **Miglitol**, they slow digestion of carbohydrate, which can lower post-meal glucose levels. They are taken with the first bite of every meal. They are not recommended for those with gastrointestinal problems as they can cause distress on the gut.

THIAZOLIDINEDIONES (TZDS)

Thizaolidinediones came on the market in 1997. They increase insulin sensitivity in muscle and fat cells. TZDs are associated with weight gain, fluid retention and exacerbation of chronic heart failure. They are taken once daily and are known as **Rosiglitazone** and **Pioglitazone**. They are not recommended for those with heart failure disease, certain types of heart disease, and the elderly. Rosiglitazone is only available through federal dispensaries.

MEGLINITIDES

Available since 1997, Meglinitides, also known as **Repaglinide** and **Nateglinide**, stimulate the beta-cells of the pancreas to produce more insulin similar to sulfonylureas. They have a shorter duration of action than sulfonylureas, are dosed three times a day and are taken with meals.

They have a risk of hypoglycemia and weight gain and are not commonly used in the U.S. as they are more costly and require a pill with every meal.

AMYLIN ANALOGS

Amylin is a hormone secreted along with insulin to help slow gastric emptying and promote earlier satiation, thus helping weight management. Amylin analogs mimic this action and have been available since 1997.

The only amylin analog is an injectable drug known as **Pramlintide**, which is approved for both T1 and T2 patients. Adverse effects are nausea and hypoglycemia.

GLUCAGON-LIKE PEPTIDE-1 (GLP-1) AGONISTS

GLP-1 agonists came on the market in 2005. Also known as incretions, GLP-1 agonists are hormones, which are released during meals from endocrine cells in your gut. They tell your pancreas to secrete insulin in the presence of hyperglycemia, but are short-lived since they are broken down by the enzyme DDP-4. Because the incretion effect is impaired in T2, GLP-1 agonists help secrete insulin without hypoglycemia.

Other beneficial effects of GLP-1 agonists are slowing gastric emptying, thus reducing the appetite and food intake.

Names of GLP-1 agonists are **Exenatide**, **Exantide XR**, **Liraglutide**, **Albiglutide** and **Dulaglutide**. They are only available as injectibles, and depending on the type, are taken once or twice per day or once per week.

Adverse effects may be mild gastrointestinal distress and nausea, which are normally short lived.

These drugs are not recommended for those with very high triglycerides or a history of pancreatitis. The American Diabetes Association recommends GLP-1 agonists as an option for second-line therapy after Metformin or in combination with Metformin.

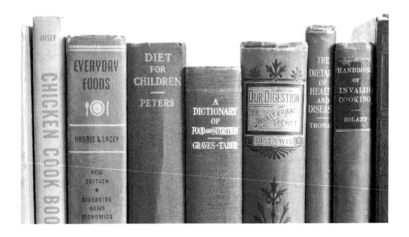

DIPEPTIDYL PEPTIDASE-4 (DDP-4) INHIBITORS

DDP-4 inhibitors entered the market in 2006. Here's how they work: your body secretes a natural hormone called an incretion, which tells your pancreas to release insulin following a meal to lower blood glucose. When incretions are released, an enzyme known as dipeptidyl pedtidase-4 (DDP-4) removes it as a normal physiological function. Some people with T2 do not make enough incretion, so the DDP-4 inhibitors help the incretion to stay in the body longer, which allows more insulin release, thus lowering blood glucose levels.

Names for DDP-4 inhibitors are **Sitagliptin**, **Saxagliptin**, **Linagliptin** and **Alogliptin** and are normally taken once per day. Many are now combined with Metformin for ease for those who need both types of medication. They have no notable side effects, but are not recommended for individuals with kidney disease.

SODIUM-GLUCOSE COTRANSPORTER 2 (SGLT-2) INHIBITORS

The newest kid on the block, SGLT-2 inhibitors, also known as glucuretics, work by increasing glucose excretion in the urine (about 80 grams per day).

They are taken once daily and can be found in combination with Metformin. Common names are **Canagliflzin**, **Dapaglifozin** and **Empaglifozin.**

They are not recommended for those prone to yeast or urinary tract infections or those with kidney disease.

If you are prone to yeast infections or are uncircumcised, there is a 10 percent risk of developing a yeast infection. Ask your provider about ways to prevent and treat a yeast infection should it occur with this medication.

INSULIN

Insulin is the therapy chosen for those with T1 and many who have T2 and GDM. Using insulin like the body would is not easy, as it needs insulin when you are not eating to balance the glucose secreted by the liver, and after you have eaten to process the meal. Insulin that is always running in the background is known as **basal insulin**. Insulin needed to process a meal is called **bolus insulin**.

If you imagine the pancreas as a sprinkler system, it can help you understand the process. When the body is in the fasting state, the sprinklers deliver a fine mist of insulin. When you eat, they open wide for a stream of insulin for a short period of time.

If someone is using an insulin pump, short acting insulin is the only type of insulin used. The pump delivers a constant dose of basal insulin (based on one's lifestyle and needs). With a meal, a bolus dose of insulin can be administered to cover the amount of carbohydrates eaten. This type of system eliminates the need for multiple insulin shots throughout the day.

Types of insulin are known as short- or fast-acting and long-acting. The first type of insulin available was in human form. Regular, also known as "**R**" and Neutral Protamine Hagerdorn, also known as "**NPH**," were prescribed in combination to create a basal/bolus effect. The R was prescribed before meals, and the NPH twice a day to assist with coverage between meals. This combination frequently resulted in frequent episodes of hypoglycemia and poor glucose control.

MYTH: Once you are diagnosed with diabetes, you will need insulin shots.

FACT: If caught early, T2 diabetes can be managed with lifestyle — diet and exercise. If more advanced, multiple oral medications exist that can control blood glucose levels. If you have diabetes, you may never need to be on insulin shots.

In 2001, pharmaceutical companies designed insulin that was better able to mimic the body's own insulin production, also known as insulin analogs.

Short-acting insulins available and given before a meal are **Lispro**, **Aspart** and **Glulisine**. They last approximately 1-3 hours and are considered bolus insulin.

Long-acting insulins available are **Glargine**, **Detemir** and **Degludec**. Glargine was designed to last 24 hours as a basal insulin and be taken once a day, but may only last 12-16 hours in some patients.

Detemir lasts approximately 12 hours and is designed to be taken twice a day. Degludec has a longer duration of approximately 30-42 hours, and is taken once daily.

A combination of background or basal insulin and bolus insulin is considered the optimal physiological insulin replacement for those on insulin therapy. Testing and patience are required to determine the mix that is appropriate for you. If you are on insulin therapy, make sure your provider is comfortable with prescribing insulin.

Sometimes insulin can be used on a short-term basis. If you a newly diagnosed with T2 and your A1C is elevated, your prescriber may use insulin to lower your glucose readings and "rest" your beta-cells until your glucose values are in a more normal range.

If your body is able to make insulin, you may be able to transition to other agents. Your doctor can order a test called a C-peptide to assess if your body is making insulin.

Nicky's
Wakeup Call

Nicky was a young patient who got a wake-up call from her doctor about diabetes. She was 15 years old when she was referred to me by her pediatrician due to insulin resistance and risk of diabetes. She decided to take matters into her own hands and control her risk factors through diet and exercise. Here is her story:

When I stepped on the scale at my doctor's office, I am sure my face was an unpleasant mix of surprise and horror. This was not the first time my weight had jumped up in a short amount of time. However, this time the numbers went too high.

My doctor said I was on the verge of diabetes. I needed to address my situation immediately and see a nutritionist who could help me see more clearly.

I am happy to say that Susan Dopart did more than just help me see. She gave me 20/20 weight management vision.

What I learned from Susan is that the insulin I produce is not sensitive enough to elicit a normal response from my liver, fat and muscle cells. I am especially sensitive to simple carbohydrates and foods like pasta, bread, and cereal, which had all been staples in my diet.

Exercise was another reason I was in such trouble. At one time, I worked out about eight hours a week as a competitive dancer, but injuries and personal reasons stopped me from continuing, and I did nothing to replace the exercise regimen.

After almost a year of the occasional workout and eating pasta for dinner most nights, it was a total shock to start running every day and to eat larger amounts of protein. I still have the occasional piece of pie, but even when I indulge I can feel the effect on my body. I used to get horrible stomachaches after eating loads of pasta or a baked potato, and did not know why. Now I know.

Since I've started treating my body the way it should be, there is no way I'll trade my "ignorance is bliss" way of life for what I know now. I sleep better. I'm able to run longer distances. I am losing weight, and I know I'm building the foundation for a healthier adulthood.

Links

ANTI-INFLAMMATORY EATING

www.susandopart.com/2010/09/lunching-for-longevity-anti-inflammatory-eating/

BEVERAGES

www.susandopart.com/2009/11/juice-equals-soda/

www.susandopart.com/2013/04/is-juicing-healthy-and-good-for-you/

www.ncbi.nlm.nih.gov/pubmed/23493538

www.susandopart.com/2010/08/beverages-and-weight-gain-you-are-what-you-drink/

www.susandopart.com/2014/09/drink-responsibly-beverage-choices-for-your-health/

www.susandopart.com/2013/06/alcohol-the-gateway-drug-to-eating/

BREAKFAST

www.ncbi.nlm.nih.gov/pubmed/25724569

www.ncbi.nlm.nih.gov/pubmed/25686619

www.ncbi.nlm.nih.gov/pubmed/25787236

www.ncbi.nlm.nih.gov/pubmed/24094031

www.susandopart.com/2011/04/protein-and-breakfast

www.susandopart.com/2012/12/dont-wait-to-prevent-diabetes-start-today-with-3-easy-ways

www.ncbi.nlm.nih.gov/pubmed/25231499

www.susandopart.com/2012/06/confused-about-carbs-5-common-myths/

www.ncbi.nlm.nih.gov/pubmed/25833777

CAFFEINE

www. susandopart.com/2011/08/coffee-insulin-resistance-and-hypoglycemia/

www.ncbi.nlm.nih.gov/pubmed/17599854

CARBOHYDRATES AND INSULIN RESISTANCE

www.susandopart.com/2014/07/are-you-carb-intolerant

www. susandopart.com/2014/05/is-it-a-carbohydrate-issue-or-a-fat-issue/

www.susandopart.com/2016/02/the-beta-cell-bank-the-false-sense-of-a-normal-glucose/

www.susandopart.com/2010/07/are-you-eating-more-carbs-than-you-think/

www.susandopart.com/2013/02/why-eating-your-broccoli-does-matter/

www.susandopart.com/2013/02/whole-grain-reality

www.susandopart.com/2010/08/whats-the-story-on-quinoa-and-protein/

www.susandopart.com/2013/10/oatmeal-cholesterol-and-insulin-resistance/

www.susandopart.com/2012/10/fat-in-your-liver/

www.susandopart.com/2014/08/insulin-the-driver-of-inflammation/

www.ncbi.nlm.nih.gov/pubmed/24962189

www.ncbi.nlm.nih.gov/pubmed/1396481

CARBOHYDRATE SUBSTITUTES

www.susandopart.com/2016/07/easy-guilt-free-pizza/

www.susandopart.com/2009/09/versatile-high-protein-lasagna/

www.susandopart.com/2010/07/alternatives-for-starches/

CONDIMENTS

www.susandopart.com/2015/04/carbs-in-your-condiments/

www.susandopart.com/2016/07/dressing-up-your-salad/

DARK CHOCOLATE

www.susandopart.com/2013/05/3-reasons-to-convert-to-dark-chocolate/

www.ncbi.nlm.nih.gov/pubmed/23254472

DIABETES DISTRESS

www.susandopart.com/2015/03/natural-ways-to-de-stress-your-immune-system/

www.ncbi.nlm.nih.gov/pubmed/25827438

EXERCISE AND ACTIVITY

www.ncbi.nlm.nih.gov/pubmed/23761134

www.susandopart.com/2014/10/stepping-up-your-exercise-game/

www.susandopart.com/2014/05/preventing-alzheimers-disease-3-strategies-to-prevent-cognitive-loss-with-age/

www.ncbi.nlm.nih.gov/pubmed/25187675

www.ncbi.nlm.nih.gov/pubmed/22875231

www.ncbi.nlm.nih.gov/pubmed/22374636

www.ncbi.nlm.nih.gov/pubmed/24773370

www.ncbi.nlm.nih.gov/pubmed/21700302

www.ncbi.nlm.nih.gov/pubmed/20044474

FASTING AND METABOLISM

www.susandopart.com/2014/01/losing-fat-the-twelve-hour-fast/

www.ncbi.nlm.nih.gov/pubmed/23637357

www.susandopart.com/2011/06/where-did-my-metabolism-go

www.susandopart.com/2013/01/does-skipping-meals-trim-your-waistline/

FIBER

www.ncbi.nlm.nih.gov/pubmed/25561122

www.ncbi.nlm.nih.gov/pubmed/24901089

FOOD DECISIONS

www.susandopart.com/2013/08/counter-the-cues-3-easy-food-decisions-to-improve-your-health/

www.susandopart.com/2013/07/over-220-food-decisions-each-day/

FRUIT

www.susandopart.com/2013/04/bananas-sugar-and-resistant-starch/

www.ncbi.nlm.nih.gov/pubmed/22815837

GROCERY SHOPPING TIPS

www.susandopart.com/2014/09/fast-food-in-the-grocery-store/

www.susandopart.com/2012/11/5-secrets-of-supermarket-shopping/

www.susandopart.com/2011/05/navigating-the-grocery-store-maze/

HEALTHY FATS

www.ncbi.nlm.nih.gov/pubmed/25460732

www.nutritionj.biomedcentral.com/articles/10.1186/1475-2891-12-155

HEALTHY GUT

www. susandopart.com/2016/01/its-all-in-your-gut-changing-your-health-for-2016/

www.susandopart.com/2016/05/change-your-metabolism-balancing-gut-hormones-food-timing-and-sleep/

www.susandopart.com/2013/05/your-gut-the-gateway-to-health/

www.susandopart.com/2012/08/strain-no-more-natural-ways-to-eliminate-constipation/

HOLIDAY AND SPECIAL OCCASION EATING

www. susandopart.com/2016/11/healthy-gluten-free-wild-rice-veggie-stuffing/

www. susandopart.com/2016/09/eggs-easter-and-spring-eating/

www.susandopart.com/2012/12/to-roll-or-not-to-roll/

www. susandopart.com/2014/10/avoiding-the-halloween-hangover/

www. susandopart.com/2010/11/tips-to-de-stress-your-holiday-season/

www.susandopart.com/2010/11/giving-thanks-after-thanksgiving/

www. susandopart.com/2015/01/superbowl-2015-food-frenzy/

www. susandopart.com/2012/02/healthy-gluten-free-valentines-day-cookie/

IMPORTANCE OF CHOLINE

www.susandopart.com/2013/09/cracking-the-code-on-eggs/

www.susandopart.com/2012/08/choline-the-next-vitamin-d/

www.ncbi.nlm.nih.gov/pubmed/25833969

INSTANT PRODUCTS AND BLOOD GLUCOSE

www.susandopart.com/2010/07/cancer-and-carbohydrates/

www.susandopart.com/2013/08/the-search-for-the-perfect-diet/

www.susandopart.com/2010/04/obesity-insulin-levels-and-cancer/

INSULIN AND BLOOD GLUCOSE MONITORING

www.ncbi.nlm.nih.gov/pubmed/24013982

www.ncbi.nlm.nih.gov/pubmed/24843694

www.ncbi.nlm.nih.gov/pubmed/25732978

LABELS

www.susandopart.com/2011/02/are-you-trapped-by-treats/

www.susandopart.com/2011/01/diabetes-prevention-love-carbs-6-steps-to-avoid-diabetes/

www.susandopart.com/2014/01/what-is-your-tolerance-for-sugar-and-sweet/

LIFESTYLE AND GLUCOSE VALUES

www.susandopart.com/2011/11/time-for-health/

www.ncbi.nlm.nih.gov/pubmed/12610028

www.susandopart.com/2015/02/3-stress-foods-to-avoid-with-autoimmune-disorders/

MEAL BALANCE AND IMPORTANCE OF PROTEIN AND HEALTHY FATS

www.susandopart.com/2012/05/6-ways-protein-helps-satiation-and-weight-loss/

www.susandopart.com/2012/04/in-defense-of-fat-7-surprising-facts/

www.susandopart.com/2014/07/are-you-carb-intolerant/

www.youtube.com/watch?v=tC_qBC1EEvw

www.susandopart.com/2010/07/is-it-healthier-to-be-vegetarian/

MINDFUL EATING

www.susandopart.com/2014/04/breaking-through-a-weight-plateau/

www.susandopart.com/2010/05/does-eckhart-tolles-power-of-now-apply-to-mindful-eating/

MOVIES AND THEATRE EATING

www.susandopart.com/2010/09/take-control-of-your-movie-theatre-experience/

www.susandopart.com/2009/11/what-about-that-movie-popcorn/

NON-NUTRITIVE SWEETENERS

www. susandopart.com/2016/06/sweeteners-the-effects-on-your-body-are-not-so-sweet/

www.susandopart.com/2010/07/sugar-or-sweetener-your-body-knows-whats-right/

www.susandopart.com/2013/12/resetting-your-taste-buds/

www.ncbi.nlm.nih.gov/pubmed/25231862

OMEGA-3-FATS

www.susandopart.com/2015/04/should-i-continue-taking-my-fish-oil

www.susandopart.com/2012/04/3-reasons-to-keep-taking-your-omega-3s

www.ncbi.nlm.nih.gov/pubmed/21593505

www.ncbi.nlm.nih.gov/pubmed/25329601

www.susandopart.com/2014/05/flax-or-chia

www.ncbi.nlm.nih.gov/pubmed/25841249

www.ncbi.nlm.nih.gov/pubmed/25180479

www.ncbi.nlm.nih.gov/pubmed/25030769

ORGANIZING YOUR FOOD

www.susandopart.com/2011/06/what-can-i-eat-for-lunch

www.susandopart.com/2010/08/organizing-your-food-world

POLYPHENOLS

www.ncbi.nlm.nih.gov/pubmed/25191617

www.ncbi.nlm.nih.gov/pubmed/26742071

PROBIOTICS

www.susandopart.com/2016/01/its-all-in-your-gut-changing-your-health-for-2016/

www.susandopart.com/2014/02/should-you-be-taking-a-probiotic/

www.ncbi.nlm.nih.gov/pubmed/25659049

SCREEN TIME

www.susandopart.com/2011/11/time-for-health/

www.ncbi.nlm.nih.gov/pubmed/12733740

SITTING AND GLUCOSE VALUES

www.susandopart.com/2015/02/sitting-is-the-new-smoking/

www.susandopart.com/2010/01/watching-tv-linked-to-higher-risk-of-heart-disease/

www.ncbi.nlm.nih.gov/pubmed/24863593

www.ncbi.nlm.nih.gov/pubmed/20650954

SLEEP

www.ncbi.nlm.nih.gov/pubmed/16983057

www.ncbi.nlm.nih.gov/pubmed/15583226

www.ncbi.nlm.nih.gov/pubmed/25715415

www.susandopart.com/2016/05/change-your-metabolism-balancing-gut-hormones-food-timing-and-sleep/

www. susandopart.com/2010/04/shrink-your-waist-with-sleep-and-protein

www.susandopart.com/2012/07/sleep-the-undervalued-lifestyle-habit/

SNACKS

www.susandopart.com/2009/04/what-about-those-snacks

www.ncbi.nlm.nih.gov/pubmed/18716179

www.ncbi.nlm.nih.gov/pubmed/18296372

SPENDING TIME IN THE KITCHEN AND GLUCOSE VALUES

www.ncbi.nlm.nih.gov/pubmed/25245799

SPICES AND APPETITE

www.ncbi.nlm.nih.gov/pubmed/22038945

STICK TO A SCHEDULE

www.ncbi.nlm.nih.gov/pubmed/25562265

SUPPLEMENTS

www.susandopart.com/2015/09/surprising-supplements-to-manage-diabetes/

www.ncbi.nlm.nih.gov/pubmed/25381809

www.ncbi.nlm.nih.gov/pubmed/17065669

www.susandopart.com/2016/02/the-beta-cell-bank-the-false-sense-of-a-normal-glucose/

www.ncbi.nlm.nih.gov/pubmed/25498346

www.ncbi.nlm.nih.gov/pubmed/18442638

www.ncbi.nlm.nih.gov/pubmed/27255472

www.susandopart.com/2013/10/healthy-alternatives-to-depression-or-anxiety-drugs-inositol-nac-and-sam-e/

www.ncbi.nlm.nih.gov/pubmed/25609734

www.ncbi.nlm.nih.gov/pubmed/12057717

www.susandopart.com/2013/02/energy-and-anti-aging-in-a-pill-coenzyme-q10-and-ubiquinol/

www.ncbi.nlm.nih.gov/pubmed/24195048

SWEETENERS AND FRUCTOSE

www.susandopart.com/2012/05/5-myths-about-everyday-foods/

www.ncbi.nlm.nih.gov/pubmed/25639270

TEA CONSUMPTION AND BLOOD GLUCOSE LEVELS

www.susandopart.com/2009/08/tea-and-aging

www.ncbi.nlm.nih.gov/pubmed/25707691

www.ncbi.nlm.nih.gov/pubmed/19723184

TRAVELING

www.susandopart.com/2012/06/vacation-eats/

www.susandopart.com/2010/07/airport-food/

USING APPS

www.susandopart.com/2015/01/an-app-a-day-keeps-the-doctor-away/

VITAMIN D

www.ncbi.nlm.nih.gov/pubmed/18377099

www.susandopart.com/2014/11/vitamin-d-vitamin-sunshine-or-hormone/

www.susandopart.com/2010/12/avoid-the-common-cold-with-these-5-easy-steps/

WEIGHT MANAGEMENT

www.susandopart.com/2014/08/when-diabetes-ignorance-is-not-bliss/

www.susandopart.com/2012/11/diabetes-prevention-its-all-about-the-beta-cells/

www.ncbi.nlm.nih.gov/pubmed/25685282

Glossary

ADRENAL GLANDS – small glands located at the top of each kidney that produce different types of hormones, including sex hormones and cortisol.

ANTIOXIDANTS – comparable to a scavenger or fire extinguisher in the body that gets rid of free radials (byproducts of normal reactions that happen like when an apple turns brown or iron turns rusty). Free radicals have the potential to cause damage to cells. Common antioxidants are vitamins C, E, and beta-carotene.

BETA-CELLS – a type of cell located in the pancreas that produces insulin. Measuring your C-peptide is a way to directly measure how much insulin your pancreas produces. If your C-peptide is low or undetectable, you will need injectable insulin. If it is normal to high and your A1C is elevated, you may need an oral medication.

CARBOHYDRATE COUNTING – counting the amount of carbohydrates one is ingesting to match your level of insulin resistance and/or insulin administration. Normally, carbohydrates are counted in units of 15 grams to match one unit of insulin, but can vary depending on insulin sensitivity.

CARBOHYDRATE INTOLERANCE – when someone has the inability to metabolize carbohydrate normally. When consuming more carbohydrate than your body can handle, the pancreas secretes an overabundance of insulin, which makes the body very efficient at storing fat.

CONTINUOUS GLUCOSE MONITOR (CGM) – a monitor that uses wireless technology to collect glucose readings from a small sensor inserted under the skin. The monitor can show readings within 1-5 minutes, and if the glucose value is out of range, alarm alerts can be programmed. A CGM also can be used to assess glucose trends and is often paired with an insulin pump.

CHROMOSOMES – structures in the body that contain the genetic information necessary to direct the functioning of all cells and systems of the body.

CHOLINE – sometimes classified as part of the vitamin B-complex, choline decreases the amount of fat in the liver. A few studies showed those with diets high in choline had less inflammatory markers in the body. Foods high in choline include egg yolks, beef, trout, salmon, tomatoes and kidney beans.

CORTISOL – a steroid hormone released by the adrenal gland that regulates carbohydrate metabolism, maintains blood pressure, and is released when an individual is under stress.

DIABETIC COMPLICATIONS – complications related to having diabetes such as neuropathy, nephropathy, and retinopathy.

DIABETIC KIDNEY DISEASE/NEPHROPATHY – a complication that occurs in some people with diabetes in which the filters of the kidney, the glomeruli, become damaged and can lead to decline in the function of the kidneys. Diabetic kidney disease can be prevented with good glycemic control, as demonstrated by the Diabetes Complication and Control Trial.

DNA – the primary carrier of genetic information, found in chromosomes.

EPIGENETICS – the environmental influence on genes beyond what is encoded in the DNA. As an example, a mother has the ability to change what happens to her child in the womb by lifestyle factors such as diet and exercise.

FIRST PHASE INSULIN – the insulin that is secreted within the first two minutes of food intake and continues for approximately 10-15 minutes. The second phase of insulin follows and continues until one's blood glucose is normalized.

FRUCTOSAMINE – like the A1C test, fructosamine is a measure of the average blood glucose values over the previous 2-3 weeks and can be used to assess insulin resistance in the early stages before an A1C is elevated.

GAD ANTIBODY TEST – a test to determine whether someone has T1 or LADA. It measures whether the body is producing a type of antibody, which lowers the function of the pancreas.

GESTATIONAL DIABETES (GDM) – a carbohydrate intolerance of variable severity with onset of the first recognition during pregnancy. GDM is a complex endocrinology disorder caused by multiple factors, especially insulin resistance.

GLUCOMETER – a monitor used for testing the blood glucose level. The glucometer measures blood glucose at a point in time. These readings change throughout the day depending on food consumed, activity and stress levels. For a comprehensive reading that shows your values all throughout the day, a CGM device will give you a more complete picture.

GLUT4 – a compound that helps the transport of glucose into the cells and is enhanced by exercise. Glut4 decreases the need for insulin by opening the door to the cells for glucose from the inside out.

GLYCEMIC INDEX – a term that measures how high a particular food raises your blood glucose level, a number between 0-100.

GLYCEMIC LOAD – a term coined by Walter Willet, MD, chairman of the Nutrition Department at Harvard Medical School of Public Health. Glycemic load indicates how much someone's blood glucose values rise in proportion to how much food he or she consumes of that particular food. For example, a food may have a high glycemic index, but if only a small portion of that food is consumed, the load is minimal.

GUT HORMONES – a group of hormones that control various functions of the digestion and are present in the stomach, pancreas and intestines.

GLYCOSYLATED HEMOGLOBIN A1C – a blood test that measures your average blood glucose over the previous three months. For those without diabetes, a normal A1C is between 4.0-5.6% depending on the laboratory. Pre-diabetes is considered 5.7-6.4% and over 6.5% for diabetes. The A1C is directly correlated to your risk of diabetic complications. If you are on diabetes medications such as sulfonylureas or insulin and are experiencing highs and lows, the A1C may not capture the picture of what is truly happening with your blood glucose values.

HYPERGLYCEMIA – the condition of having a blood glucose level above normal range (more than 130 mg/dl). Food, medications, lack of sleep and illness can all contribute to raising your blood glucose values.

HYPOGLYCEMIA – the condition of having a blood glucose value below normal range (normally less than 70 in both T1 and T2 diabetes, but less than 50 in GDM). Those experiencing a low glucose may feel light-headed, shaky and sweaty. In many cases, low glucose values can be a result of medications such as too much insulin given. If hypoglycemia is a result of medications, it can be a medical emergency and need to be treated with glucose and/or food immediately. When a person experiences what is known as reactive hypoglycemia (when the body tries to readjust from a high glucose), it is not an emergency, but food cravings may develop and many compensate with extra food.

INSULIN – a hormone produced by the beta-cells in the pancreas that allows glucose to enter the cells for energy. During pregnancy and commonly with a diagnosis of diabetes, it may be necessary to take insulin shots to normalize blood glucose values. Insulin is not addictive and can be used for the short-term to lower blood glucose values. Insulin is necessary for people with T1 diabetes, as well as those who have T2 diabetes whose pancreas has exceeded its capacity to compensate and/or can no longer produce sufficient insulin.

INSULIN PUMP – a computerized device that delivers short-acting insulin through a catheter placed under the skin. Pumps can be programmed to deliver insulin based on one's glucose levels and carbohydrate intake to deliver varying rates of basal and bolus insulin throughout the 24 hours based on needs.

INSULIN SENSITIVE – those with a normal metabolism in which the body responds to smaller amounts of insulin to lower blood glucoses levels.

INSULIN RESISTANCE – a condition that occurs when the body doesn't respond normally to the insulin the pancreas is producing. As a result, it is harder for glucose to enter the cells.

ISLET CELLS – clusters of cells located in the pancreas that produce hormones.

LADA (LATENT AUTOIMMUNE DIABETES IN ADULTS) – a slowly developing kind of T1 diabetes in which the cells of the pancreas stop producing as much insulin as they once did. The loss of beta-cells is more gradual than in T1 and can take several years before insulin is required. LADA is commonly misdiagnosed as T2. If suspected, blood tests known as C-peptide and antibodies for GAD and islet cells should be checked. A diagnosis of LADA requires antibodies that are elevated along with a low C-peptide.

MACRONUTRIENTS – a term that refers to the three main components of food: carbohydrate, protein and fat.

METFORMIN – an oral medication that assists in lowering blood glucose by lowering the amount of glucose discharged by the liver, thereby increasing the body's response to its own insulin and lowering the amount of glucose absorbed from food.

MODY (MATURITY ONSET DIABETES OF THE YOUNG) – this type of diabetes is most likely due to genetics and affects 1-2 percent of individuals with diabetes; it normally develops before the age of 25. MODY is caused by a change in a single gene and six types have been identified. MODY needs to be managed, but does not normally require insulin.

NEUROPATHY – damage to the nerves that occurs as a result of diabetes, thought to be the result of prolonged elevated levels of blood glucose. Neuropathy can be prevented.

NON-ALCOHOLIC FATTY LIVER DISEASE (NAFLD) – characterized by fatty deposits in the liver, which can lead to cirrhosis. The exact cause is not known, but a high intake of sugars, especially fructose, is associated with an increased incidence.

OMEGA-3-FATS – three types of fats known as ALA, DHA and EPA, which lower inflammation in the body and assist in providing important nutrients for the cells in the body and brain. DHA is particularly important for development of the brain in utero.

PANCREAS – an organ that serves both as an endocrine gland that produces hormones (including insulin), and a digestive organ that produces enzymes necessary for digestion of food.

POLYPHENOLS – the most abundant antioxidants in the diet, coming mostly from fruit, tea, cocoa, walnuts and flaxseeds. Polyphenols have numerous health benefits including prevention of degenerative diseases such as cancer and heart disease.

PROINSULIN – a building block for insulin that is made by the pancreas. Measuring proinsulin in the blood can assist with figuring out the potential risk for T1 or T2 diabetes, as well as risk of coronary artery disease.

RESISTANT STARCH – starch in the diet that is resistant to digestion since it functions like a fiber. Resistant starch is present in unripe bananas, some grains, seeds and legumes.

RETINOPATHY – damage to the retina in the eye caused by complications of diabetes, which eventually can lead to blindness. Retinopathy is preventable with good diabetes care, which includes an annual eye exam and blood glucose normalization. Avoid weight-bearing exercise if your blood glucose values are above 250-300 mg/dl., as it can result in complications to the small vessels in the eyes.

STACKING – is a term referring to "stacking" insulin when one administers more than one correction of insulin within the same period that insulin has already been given. Stacking can lead to hypoglycemia and more highs and lows in blood glucose values.

TELOMERES – DNA complexes on the ends of chromosomes. As one ages, telomeres shorten. Studies reveal stress and lifestyle choices have been linked to telomere length.

TEST STRIPS – disposable strips the glucometer reads and uses to calculate blood glucose values.

TYPE 1 DIABETES (T1) – formerly known as juvenile-onset diabetes but can develop even in geriatric adults, in which the beta-cells of the pancreas stop insulin production, requiring life-long insulin administration. The exact cause is not known, but research indicates a possible genetic link triggered by a virus.

TYPE 2 DIABETES (T2) – formerly known as adult-onset diabetes but can develop even in young children, characterized by insulin resistance in which the tissues of the body have less insulin sensitivity and a carbohydrate intolerance. T2 can be genetic and/or brought on by lifestyle. T2 diabetes is treated with diet and exercise/activity. If glucose values are not normalized with lifestyle interventions, medications are available that help impact glucose control.

TRIGLYCERIDES – the storage form of fat in the blood associated with carbohydrate sensitivity and insulin resistance. Alcohol intake can dramatically increase triglyceride levels.

VITAMIN D – a hormone that regulates multiple functions in the body and in utero, including bone health, brain development, immunity and insulin resistance.

Closing Thoughts

---

*Thank you for taking the time to read **101 Ways to Control your Diabetes**. The fact that you have read this book shows you care about your health. Although diabetes is a serious medical diagnosis, it does not need to have detrimental consequences. Lifestyle management for diabetes can lead to improvements in your health. With the ideas in this book, I hope you now have more ways to guide your everyday choices along a positive path.*

Knowledge is power -- use it for continued health and happiness on your journey. I wish you all the best.

Susan

A NOTE TO READERS

The information in this book is not intended or implied to be a substitute for professional medical advice, diagnoses or treatment. All content in these pages -- including text, charts, illustrations, graphics and photographs -- is for general purposes only.

You are encouraged to confirm any information obtained in or through this book with other sources, and to review all information regarding any medical condition or treatment with your physical or healthcare professional.

Never disregard professional medical advice, forego or delay seeking medical treatment because of something you have read in this book.

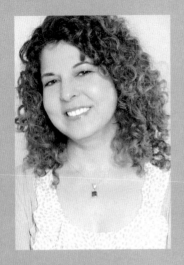

Susan B. Dopart, MS, RD, CDE, is a health, wellness, and fitness consultant who has been in private practice for more than 20 years. Susan specializes in child and adult medical nutrition related issues associated with insulin resistance, diabetes and endocrinology, cancer, PCOS and exercise. Before establishing her own practice, Susan worked at UCLA as both a medical and kidney dietitian.

She has written and contributed to multiple publications, including *The Huffington Post, SELF Maga-zine, UCLA Medicine, Sports and Cardiovascular Nutritionists SCAN, Best Life, Men's Health, Diabetes Health and Diabetes Forecast.*

After receiving her bachelor of science degree in nutrition and clinical dietetics from UC Berkeley, Susan earned a master of science degree in exercise physiology and sports medicine from California State University, Hayward. She is a certified diabetes educator (CDE).

Susan is the author of *A Recipe for Life by the Doctor's Dietitian*; *Healthy You, Healthy Baby: A Mother's Guide to Gestational Diabetes*; and *A Healthy Baker's Dozen*.

Susan is from New Jersey and grew up in Northern California before moving to Los Angeles. She resides in Santa Monica with her husband Jeffrey and canine son, Perry.

Connect online with her at susandopart.com or diabetes101health.com